THE *Skinny*
BLEND ▸ *ACTIVE*
LEAN BODY
YOGA WORKOUT PLAN

 CookNation

THE SKINNY BLEND ACTIVE
LEAN BODY YOGA WORKOUT PLAN
CALORIE COUNTED SMOOTHIES WITH GENTLE YOGA WORKOUTS FOR HEALTH & WELLBEING.

ISBN 978-1-911219-47-7

A CIP catalogue record of this book is available from the British Library

• •

DISCLAIMER

This book is designed to provide information on smoothies and juices that can be made in the Breville Blend Active and other personal blender appliances, results may differ if alternative devices are used.

BREVILLE is a trademark of Breville Pty Ltd. Bell & Mackenzie Publishing is not affiliated with the owner of the trademark and is not an authorized distributor of the trademark owner's products or services. This publication has not been prepared, approved, or licensed by Breville Pty.

Breville were not involved in the recipe development or testing of any of the recipes on this book.

A basic level of fitness is required to perform the workouts in this book. Any health concerns should be discussed with a health professional before embarking on any of the exercises detailed.

Some recipes may contain nuts or traces of nuts. Those suffering from any allergies associated with nuts should avoid any recipes containing nuts or nut based oils. This information is provided and sold with the knowledge that the publisher and author do not offer any legal or other professional advice.

In the case of a need for any such expertise consult with the appropriate professional.

This book does not contain all information available on the subject, and other sources of recipes are available.

This book has not been created to be specific to any individual's requirements.

Every effort has been made to make this book as accurate as possible. However, there may be typographical and or content errors. Therefore, this book should serve only as a general guide and not as the ultimate source of subject information.

This book contains information that might be dated and is intended only to educate and entertain.

The author and publisher shall have no liability or responsibility to any person or entity regarding any loss or damage incurred, or alleged to have incurred, directly or indirectly, by the information contained in this book.

CONTENTS

UNDER 400 CALORIES

YOGA WORKOUTS

OTHER COOKNATION TITLES

INTRODUCTION

Personal blending is the fastest way to create super-healthy, delicious single serving smoothies, juices, breakfast drinks, protein & nutrition shakes.

This no-fuss approach to a healthier way of living is a great way to increase your fruit intake, compliment your daily workouts, manage your diet and have fun making great tasting drinks.

Blend & Go devices are hugely popular especially for the health conscious and those with a busy lifestyle. Using the Blend Active couldn't be simpler…just add the ingredients as per our recipes, blend in the sports bottle then replace the blade with the leak proof lid and you're done!

All the recipes in this book have been tested using the Breville Blend Active Personal Blender but they can be used for any of the personal blenders on the market. The Breville Blend Active is a great single server blender. The most popular version comes with 2 x 600ml sports bottles with a one-touch blend button. The base unit is small, easy to clean and the blade is even strong enough to crush ice.

Adopting personal blending into your daily routine has enormous health benefits. Balancing your diet with healthy nutritious drinks can help you lose weight as part of a calorie controlled diet, boost your immune system and help fight a number of ailments. Each of the recipes in this book are calorie counted making it easy for you to keep track of your calorific intake and help you achieve your 5-A-Day quota.

Using our recipes and workouts on a daily basis, together with an overall healthy eating plan will help you feel brighter, rejuvenated, more focused and energetic.

Our delicious calorie counted smoothies and yoga workouts are a healthy combination which will set you on the path to enhanced well being.

THE YOGA PLAN WORKOUTS

Yoga is an ancient form of exercise that focuses on strength, flexibility and breathing. Originating in India more than 5,000 years ago, yoga is practiced to boost physical & mental wellbeing and has been adopted by cultures around the world. It is a safe and effective way to increase physical activity, especially strength, flexibility and balance.

Yoga is thought to have many healing properties and is beneficial for people with high blood pressure, heart disease, aches and pains, depression and stress. There are a number of different types of yoga which are generally practiced including Hatha, Vinyasa & Iyengar to name just three. The routines which have been developed for this book are not confined to one type of yoga and will give you a basic introduction to this wonderful form of exercise.

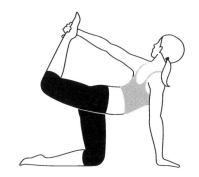

You will find three yoga workouts in this book. The first 2 routines will take around 15 minutes to complete. The third is a 30 minute relaxation session. Incorporating a yoga routine into your daily life will benefit you both physically and mentally. All you need to get started is a mat, a block and pillows for support (for the relaxation routine at the end). That said there is no need to run out and buy any equipment at all. You can do any of these routines comfortably on a rug or carpet and the yoga block can be substituted for a small strong shoe sized box.

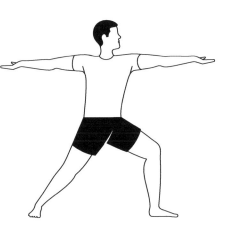

Yoga will, in time, help you 'still' your mind. When you are doing the routines try to empty your brain of any thoughts. That is not as easy as it sounds, but have patience with yourself. If you try to anchor your thoughts around your breathing you will learn to calm your mind and move towards a stillness which will benefit your well-being.

Enjoy your yoga journey.

YOGA TIPS

- A few things to remember:
- Yoga should never be approached as a competitive sport. It is a personal journey. Always listen to your body and never push yourself too hard. Concentrating on breathing is an extremely important part of yoga practice and you will learnt to use the rhythm of your breathing to help you move through the poses.
- Always move into poses on a breath exhalation and make sure you move slowly and methodically.

BLENDER TIPS

Personal blenders are simple and easy to use. Follow these tips to get the most from your device:

- When using ice in your drink, always immerse the ice first in a little liquid. You can do this in the sports bottle with the liquid ingredients you are using such as a little water or fruit juice.
- When you are adding ingredients don't fill the sports bottle above the 600ml mark (or 300ml if you use are the 300ml bottles).
- If some ingredients become stuck around the blade just detach the bottle from the base unit and give it a good shake to loosen the ingredients then blend again.

- Clean the blender base unit with a damp cloth. The blade, bottle and cap can all be placed in a dishwasher or alternatively wash with warm soapy water. For best results wash parts immediately after using.
- For stubborn ingredients that may have stuck to the blade or the inside of the bottle, half fill the bottle with warm water and a drop or two of detergent, fit the blade and attach to the base unit pulsing for 10 seconds or so.
- Use the freshest produce available. We recommend buying organic produce whenever you can if your budget allows. You can also freeze your fruit to preserve it.
- Wash your fruit and veg before blending to remove any traces of bacteria, pesticides and insects.
- Chop ingredients, especially harder produce, into small pieces to ensure smoother blending.
- Substitute where you need to. If you can't source a particular ingredient, try another instead. Experiment and enjoy!

ABOUT 🍎 CookNation

CookNation is the leading publisher of innovative and practical recipe books for the modern, health conscious cook. CookNation titles bring together delicious, easy and practical recipes with their unique approach - easy and delicious, no-nonsense recipes - making cooking for diets and healthy eating fast, simple and fun.

With a range of #1 best-selling titles - from the innovative 'Skinny' calorie-counted series, to the 5:2 Diet Recipes collection - CookNation recipe books prove that 'Diet' can still mean 'Delicious'!

THE *Skinny*

BLEND ▸ ACTIVE

LEAN BODY
YOGA WORKOUT PLAN

SMOOTHIES & JUICES UNDER 200 CALORIES

CINNAMON BERRY JUICE

185 calories per serving

Ingredients

- 1 banana
- 100g/3½oz strawberries
- 50g/2oz raspberries
- 50g/2oz fresh pineapple
- ½ tsp ground cinnamon
- Water

Method

1 Rinse all the ingredients well.

2 Peel the banana and break into small pieces.

3 Add all the fruit & vegetables to the bottle, making sure the ingredients do not go past the 600ml/20oz line on your bottle.

4 Add water, again being careful not to exceed the MAX line.

5 Twist on the blade and blend until smooth.

CHEFS NOTE
Fresh or tinned pineapple will work just as well. Use a little of the juice in place of water if you like.

RASPBERRY ALMOND SMOOTHIE

165 calories per serving

Ingredients

- 1 handful of spinach
- 1 carrot
- 200g/7oz raspberries
- 250ml/1 cup almond milk
- Water

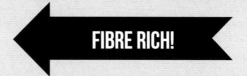

FIBRE RICH!

Method

1 Rinse all the ingredients well.

2 Remove any thick, hard stems from the spinach and roughly chop.

3 Top, tail, peel & chop the carrot.

4 Add the vegetables, fruit & almond milk to the bottle, making sure the ingredients do not go past the 600ml/20oz line on your bottle.

5 Top up with water if needed, again being careful not to exceed the MAX line.

6 Twist on the blade and blend until smooth.

CHEFS NOTE
Strawberries are also good in this lovely smoothie blend.

PAPAYA & BANANA JUICE

195 calories per serving

Ingredients

- 1 banana
- 1 papaya fruit
- 1 kiwi
- Water

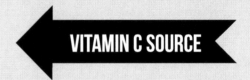
VITAMIN C SOURCE

Method

1 Rinse all the ingredients well.

2 Peel the banana and break into small pieces.

3 Peel and chop the kiwi.

4 Scoop out the papaya flesh, discarding the seeds and rind.

5 Add the fruit to the bottle, making sure the ingredients do not go past the 600ml/20oz line on your bottle.

6 Top up with water, again being careful not to exceed the MAX line.

7 Twist on the blade and blend until smooth.

CHEFS NOTE

Native to tropical America, papayas are also known as paw-paws. They are sweet & juicy with a similar taste to peaches.

ICED CHERRY JUICE

170
calories per
serving

Ingredients

- 1 handful of spinach
- 1 apple
- 150g/5oz cherries
- Handful of Ice
- Water

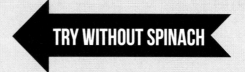

TRY WITHOUT SPINACH

Method

1 Rinse all the ingredients well.

2 Remove any thick, hard stems from the spinach and roughly chop.

3 Peel, core and chop the apple.

4 Pit the cherries and remove the stalks.

5 Add the vegetables & fruit to the bottle, making sure the ingredients do not go past the 600ml/20oz line on your bottle.

6 Top up with water and a few ice cubes, again being careful not to exceed the MAX line.

7 Twist on the blade and blend until smooth.

CHEFS NOTE
Frozen cherries are also a good option for this juice and make it even quicker to prepare.

FRUITY SPICED PINEAPPLE JUICE

SERVES 1

110 calories per serving

Ingredients

- 1 handful of spinach
- 200g/7oz pineapple chunks
- ½ red chilli
- Water

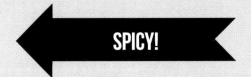

SPICY!

Method

1 Rinse all the ingredients well.

2 Remove any thick, hard stems from the spinach and roughly chop.

3 De-seed the chilli and finely chop.

4 Add the vegetables, fruit & chopped chilli to the bottle, making sure the ingredients do not go past the 600ml/20oz line on your bottle.

5 Top up with water, again being careful not to exceed the MAX line.

6 Twist on the blade and blend until smooth.

CHEFS NOTE

Use a little cayenne pepper if you don't have fresh chillies to hand.

APPLE GREENS JUICE

185 calories per serving

Ingredients

- 200g/7oz tenderstem broccoli/broccolini
- 1 apple
- 1 carrot
- Water

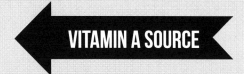
VITAMIN A SOURCE

Method

1 Rinse all the ingredients well.

2 Chop the broccoli.

3 Peel, core & chop the apple.

4 Top, tail, peel and chop the carrot.

5 Add the vegetables & fruit to the bottle, making sure the ingredients do not go past the 600ml/20oz line on your bottle.

6 Top up with water, again being careful not to exceed the MAX line.

7 Twist on the blade and blend until smooth.

CHEFS NOTE
Purple sprouting broccoli stems are a great seasonal ingredient.

ASPARAGUS & APPLE JUICE

155 calories per serving

Ingredients

- 150g/5oz asparagus tips
- 1 apple
- ½ cucumber
- Water

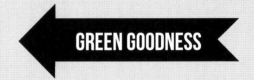
GREEN GOODNESS

Method

1 Rinse all the ingredients well.

2 Chop the asparagus tips.

3 Peel, core & chop the apple.

4 Peel & chop the cucumber.

5 Add the vegetables & fruit to the bottle, making sure the ingredients do not go past the 600ml/20oz line on your bottle.

6 Top up with water, again being careful not to exceed the MAX line.

7 Twist on the blade and blend until smooth.

CHEFS NOTE
This is a really simple juice, add an extra chopped apple if you want a sweeter taste.

PEAR PICK UP JUICE

170
calories per
serving

Ingredients

- 1 pear
- 1 apple
- 2 tsp grated fresh ginger root
- 2 tsp lemon juice
- Water

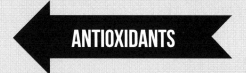

ANTIOXIDANTS

Method

1 Rinse all the ingredients well.

2 Peel, core and chop the pear & apple.

3 Add the fruit, vegetables, ginger & lemon juice to the bottle, making sure the ingredients do not go past the 600ml/20oz line on your bottle.

4 Top up with water, again being careful not to exceed the MAX line.

5 Twist on the blade and blend until smooth.

CHEFS NOTE
Adjust the freshly grated ginger to suit your own taste.

FRUIT VITAMIN C+ JUICE

180 calories per serving

Ingredients

- 1 orange
- 1 banana
- 1 tbsp lemon juice
- Water

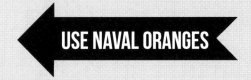

USE NAVAL ORANGES

Method

1 Rinse all the ingredients well.

2 Peel and chop the orange, discard the rind.

3 Peel the banana and break into small pieces.

4 Add the fruit, vegetables & lemon juice to the bottle, making sure the ingredients do not go past the 600ml/20oz line on your bottle.

5 Top up with water, again being careful not to exceed the MAX line.

6 Twist on the blade and blend until smooth.

CHEFS NOTE
Orange is the classic Vitamin C provider.

SUPER SALAD JUICE

45 calories per serving

Ingredients

- 1 handful of spinach
- 2 celery stalks
- 1 vine ripened tomato
- ½ cucumber
- ½ tsp cayenne pepper (optional)
- Water

Method

1 Rinse all the ingredients well.

2 Remove any thick, hard stems from the spinach and roughly chop.

3 Chop the celery, discarding any tops.

4 Chop the tomato. Peel & chop the cucumber.

5 Add the chopped salad & cayenne pepper to the bottle, making sure the ingredients do not go past the 600ml/20oz line on your bottle.

6 Top up with water, again being careful not to exceed the MAX line.

7 Twist on the blade and blend until smooth.

CHEFS NOTE

This is a really light juice, great for fresh summer mornings.

CLEANSING APPLE JUICE

110 calories per serving

Ingredients

- 1 apple
- 1 cucumber
- 1 tbsp lime juice
- Water

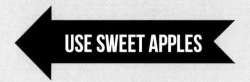
USE SWEET APPLES

Method

1 Rinse all the ingredients well.

2 Peel, core & chop the apple.

3 Peel & chop the cucumber.

4 Add the chopped fruit, vegetables & lime juice to the bottle, making sure the ingredients do not go past the 600ml/20oz line on your bottle.

5 Top up with water, again being careful not to exceed the MAX line.

6 Twist on the blade and blend until smooth.

CHEFS NOTE
Put some of the cucumber to one side if you can't fit it all in.

COCONUT CHIA JUICE

180 calories per serving

Ingredients

- 1 handful of spinach
- 1 apple
- 2 tsp chia seeds
- 250ml/1 cup coconut water
- Water

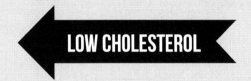

LOW CHOLESTEROL

Method

1 Rinse all the ingredients well.

2 Remove any thick, hard stems from the spinach and roughly chop.

3 Peel, core & chop the apple.

4 Add the chopped fruit, vegetables, chia seeds & coconut water to the bottle, making sure the ingredients do not go past the 600ml/20oz line on your bottle.

5 Top up with water if it needs it, again being careful not to exceed the MAX line.

6 Twist on the blade and blend until smooth.

CHEFS NOTE
Chia seeds are a great source of Vitamin B.

DOUBLE PEAR & PAK CHOI JUICE

185 calories per serving

Ingredients

- 1 pak choi/bok choy
- 2 pears
- ½ banana
- Water

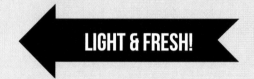

LIGHT & FRESH!

Method

1 Rinse all the ingredients well.

2 Shred the pak choi, remove any hard bulb parts.

3 Peel, core & chop the pears.

4 Peel the banana then break into small pieces.

5 Add the chopped fruit & vegetables to the bottle, making sure the ingredients do not go past the 600ml/20oz line on your bottle.

6 Top up with water, again being careful not to exceed the MAX line.

7 Twist on the blade and blend until smooth.

CHEFS NOTE
Pak choi is a great juice alternative to spinach and kale.

APPLE & LEMON JUICE

115 calories per serving

Ingredients

- 2 handfuls of spinach
- 1 apple
- 1 tbsp lemon juice
- Water

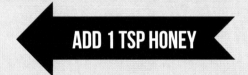
ADD 1 TSP HONEY

Method

1 Rinse all the ingredients well.

2 Remove any thick, hard stems from the spinach and roughly chop.

3 Peel, core and chop the apple.

4 Add the fruit, vegetables & lemon juice to the bottle, making sure the ingredients do not go past the 600ml/20oz line on your bottle.

5 Top up with water, again being careful not to exceed the MAX line.

6 Twist on the blade and blend until smooth.

CHEFS NOTE
Give the bottle a good shake mid-way through blending if you find all the ingredients aren't coming together.

GREEN DETOX JUICE

85
calories per
serving

Ingredients

- 1 handful of spinach
- 1 handful of kale
- 1 pear
- 1 tbsp lemon juice
- Water

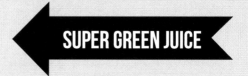
SUPER GREEN JUICE

Method

1 Rinse all the ingredients well.

2 Remove any thick, hard stems from the spinach and kale & roughly chop.

3 Peel, core and chop the pear.

4 Add the fruit, vegetables & lemon juice to the bottle, making sure the ingredients do not go past the 600ml/20oz line on your bottle.

5 Top up with water, again being careful not to exceed the MAX line.

6 Twist on the blade and blend until smooth.

CHEFS NOTE

Add a teaspoon of honey if you struggle with the taste of some of the kale based juices.

MULTI GREEN JUICE

115 calories per serving

Ingredients

- 1 handful of spinach
- 1 handful of pak choi/bok choi
- 1 apple
- Water

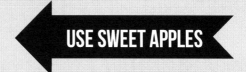

USE SWEET APPLES

Method

1 Rinse all the ingredients well.

2 Remove any thick, hard stems from the spinach & pak choi and roughly chop.

3 Peel, core and chop the apple.

4 Add the fruit & vegetables to the bottle, making sure the ingredients do not go past the 600ml/20oz line on your bottle.

5 Top up with water, again being careful not to exceed the MAX line.

6 Twist on the blade and blend until smooth.

CHEFS NOTE

Pak choi is an Asian style cabbage which is now widely available in most stores.

SUPER SALAD JUICE

55 calories per serving

Ingredients

- 2 celery stalks
- 2 vine ripened tomatoes
- ½ cucumber
- 2 tsp Worcestershire sauce (optional)
- Water

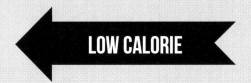
LOW CALORIE

Method

1 Rinse all the ingredients well.

2 Chop the celery, discarding any tops.

3 Chop the tomatoes. Peel & chop the cucumber.

4 Add the chopped salad & Worcestershire sauce to the bottle, making sure the ingredients do not go past the 600ml/20oz line on your bottle.

5 Top up with water, again being careful not to exceed the MAX line.

6 Twist on the blade and blend until smooth.

CHEFS NOTE
This is not a completely smooth juice, but that's not a problem. Just drink the 'bits'!

INDIAN SUMMER JUICE

135 calories per serving

Ingredients

- 1 handful of spinach
- 1 apple
- 1 carrot
- ½ tsp ground turmeric
- Water

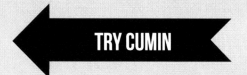

TRY CUMIN

Method

1 Rinse all the ingredients well.

2 Remove any thick, hard stems from the spinach and roughly chop.

3 Peel, core and chop the apple.

4 Top, tail, peel and chop the carrot.

5 Add the vegetables, fruit & turmeric to the bottle, making sure the ingredients do not go past the 600ml/20oz line on your bottle.

6 Top up with water, again being careful not to exceed the MAX line.

7 Twist on the blade and blend until smooth.

CHEFS NOTE
Turmeric adds colour and spice to this unusual juice. Try a pinch of cayenne pepper too.

CRISP LETTUCE & CARROT JUICE

170
calories per serving

Ingredients

- 1 baby gem lettuce
- 1 apple
- 2 carrots
- Water

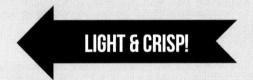
LIGHT & CRISP!

Method

1 Rinse all the ingredients well.

2 Roughly chop the lettuce and discard the heart.

3 Peel, core and cube the apple.

4 Top, tail, peel and chop the carrots.

5 Add the vegetables & fruit to the bottle, making sure the ingredients do not go past the 600ml/20oz line on your bottle.

6 Top up with water, again being careful not to exceed the MAX line.

7 Twist on the blade and blend until smooth.

CHEFS NOTE
This simple juice is packed with vitamin A.

THE *Skinny*

BLEND ▸ ACTIVE

LEAN BODY
YOGA WORKOUT PLAN

SMOOTHIES & JUICES UNDER 300 CALORIES

VERY BERRY JUICE

220
calories per serving

Ingredients

- 200g/7oz mixed berries
- 1 banana
- 1 tsp honey
- Water

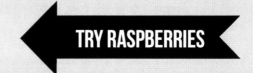
TRY RASPBERRIES

Method

1 Rinse all the ingredients well.

2 Peel the banana and break into small pieces.

3 Add the fruit and honey to the bottle, making sure the ingredients do not go past the 600ml/20oz line on your bottle.

4 Top up with water, again being careful not to exceed the MAX line.

5 Twist on the blade and blend until smooth.

CHEFS NOTE
Frozen mixed berries are a handy ingredient for this simple smoothie.

HONEYED FIG SMOOTHIE

270 calories per serving

Ingredients

- 1 banana
- 3 dried figs
- 250ml/1 cup soya milk
- 2 tsp honey
- Water

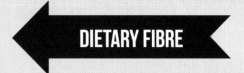

DIETARY FIBRE

Method

1 Peel the banana and break into small pieces.

2 Chop the figs.

3 Add the fruit, milk & honey to the bottle, making sure the ingredients do not go past the 600ml/20oz line on your bottle.

4 Top up with water if it needs it, again being careful not to exceed the MAX line.

5 Twist on the blade and blend until smooth.

CHEFS NOTE

Soak the dried figs for half an hour in a little warm water before chopping.

FRESH CHERRY & BANANA SMOOTHIE

260 calories per serving

Ingredients

- 200g/7oz fresh cherries
- 1 banana
- 250ml/1 cup almond milk
- Water

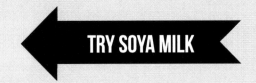
TRY SOYA MILK

Method

1 Rinse all the ingredients well.

2 De-stone, de-stalk and chop the cherries.

3 Peel the banana and break into small pieces.

4 Add the fruit & milk to the bottle, making sure the ingredients do not go past the 600ml/20oz line on your bottle.

5 Top up with water if it needs it, again being careful not to exceed the MAX line.

6 Twist on the blade and blend until smooth.

CHEFS NOTE
Fresh cherries are fabulous when they are in season but frozen cherries will work too if that's all you can get your hands on.

KIWI & SOYA MILK SMOOTHIE

295 calories per serving

Ingredients

- 2 kiwis
- 1 banana
- 250ml/1 cup soya milk
- Water

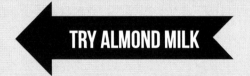
TRY ALMOND MILK

Method

1 Peel and chop the kiwis.

2 Peel the banana and break into small pieces.

3 Add the fruit & milk to the bottle, making sure the ingredients do not go past the 600ml/20oz line on your bottle.

4 Top up with water if it needs it, again being careful not to exceed the MAX line.

5 Twist on the blade and blend until smooth.

CHEFS NOTE
Use ripe kiwis to make the most of their natural sweetness.

SPINACH & PEAR SMOOTHIE

290 calories per serving

Ingredients

- 1 handful spinach
- 1 banana
- 1 pear
- 1 cup/250ml semi skimmed milk

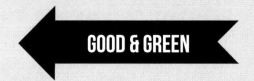

GOOD & GREEN

Method

1 Remove any thick, hard stems from the spinach and roughly chop.

2 Peel the banana and break into small pieces

3 Peel, core and chop the pear.

4 Add the fruit, vegetables & milk to the bottle, making sure the ingredients do not go past the 600ml/20oz line on your bottle.

5 Twist on the blade and blend until smooth.

CHEFS NOTE
Try using a fresh peach in place of the pear.

PINEAPPLE ICE CRUSH

205 calories per serving

Ingredients

- 1 apple
- 200g/7oz pineapple chunks
- Handful of ice cubes
- Water

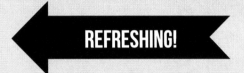

REFRESHING!

Method

1 Rinse all the ingredients well.

2 Peel, core and chop the apple.

3 Add the fruit to the bottle, making sure the ingredients do not go past the 600ml/20oz line on your bottle.

4 Top up with the ice and water, again being careful not to exceed the MAX line.

5 Twist on the blade and blend until smooth.

CHEFS NOTE
Pineapple is a great source of manganese and vitamin C.

FRESH HERB JUICE

215
calories per
serving

Ingredients

- 1 handful of spinach
- 2 tbsp chopped of fresh mint
- 2 tbsp chopped of fresh basil
- 2 apples
- Water

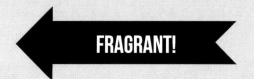

FRAGRANT!

Method

1 Rinse all the ingredients well.

2 Remove any thick, hard stems from the spinach and roughly chop.

3 Peel, core and chop the apples.

4 Add the fruit, vegetables & herbs to the bottle, making sure the ingredients do not go past the 600ml/20oz line on your bottle.

5 Top up with water, again being careful not to exceed the MAX line.

6 Twist on the blade and blend until smooth.

CHEFS NOTE
You can experiment with whichever mix of fresh herbs you prefer.

ALMOND & PINEAPPLE JUICE

260 calories per serving

Ingredients

- 1 handful of spinach
- 1 banana
- 200g/7oz pineapple chunks
- 1 tbsp ground almonds
- Water

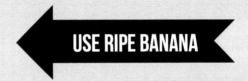
USE RIPE BANANA

Method

1 Rinse all the ingredients well.

2 Remove any thick, hard stems from the spinach and roughly chop.

3 Peel the banana and break into small pieces.

4 Add the fruit, vegetables & ground almonds to the bottle, making sure the ingredients do not go past the 600ml/20oz line on your bottle.

5 Top up with water, again being careful not to exceed the MAX line.

6 Twist on the blade and blend until smooth.

CHEFS NOTE
Try using almond milk in place of water as the base for this blend.

PARSLEY & APPLE JUICE

210
calories per
serving

Ingredients

- 1 handful of spinach
- 2 apples
- 2 tbsp chopped flat leaf parsley
- 1 tbsp lemon juice
- Water

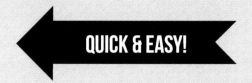

QUICK & EASY!

Method

1 Rinse all the ingredients well.

2 Remove any thick, hard stems from the spinach and roughly chop.

3 Peel, core and chop the apples.

4 Add the fruit, vegetables, parsley & lemon juice to the bottle, making sure the ingredients do not go past the 600ml/20oz line on your bottle.

5 Top up with water, again being careful not to exceed the MAX line.

6 Twist on the blade and blend until smooth.

CHEFS NOTE
Flat leaf parsley works better than the curly variety for this juice.

PINEAPPLE PEPPER JUICE

260 calories per serving

Ingredients

- 1 orange pepper
- 1 banana
- 200g/7oz pineapple chunks
- Water

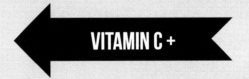

VITAMIN C +

Method

1 Rinse all the ingredients well.

2 De-seed and chop the pepper.

3 Peel the banana and break into small pieces.

4 Add the fruit & vegetables to the bottle, making sure the ingredients do not go past the 600ml/20oz line on your bottle.

5 Top up with water, again being careful not to exceed the MAX line.

6 Twist on the blade and blend until smooth.

CHEFS NOTE

Use whichever peppers you have to hand but avoid green peppers as they tend to be a little bitter in juice blends.

CALYPSO JUICE

250 calories per serving

Ingredients

- 1 handful of spinach
- 1 banana
- 200g/7oz pineapple chunks
- 250ml/1 cup coconut water
- Water

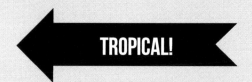 TROPICAL!

Method

1 Rinse all the ingredients well.

2 Remove any thick, hard stems from the spinach and roughly chop.

3 Peel the banana and break into small pieces.

4 Add the fruit, vegetables & coconut water to the bottle, making sure the ingredients do not go past the 600ml/20oz line on your bottle.

5 Top up with water if it needs it, again being careful not to exceed the MAX line.

6 Twist on the blade and blend until smooth.

CHEFS NOTE
Coconut water is a great juice ingredient with low levels of fat, carbohydrates, and calories.

SKINNY GREEN JUICE

230 calories per serving

Ingredients

- 2 apples
- 1 courgette/zucchini
- ½ cucumber
- Water

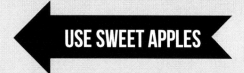

USE SWEET APPLES

Method

1 Rinse all the ingredients well.

2 Peel, core and chop the apples.

3 Peel the courgette and cucumber. Top & tail them both before chopping.

4 Add the vegetables & fruit to the bottle, making sure the ingredients do not go past the 600ml/20oz line on your bottle.

5 Top up with water, again being careful not to exceed the MAX line.

6 Twist on the blade and blend until smooth.

CHEFS NOTE
This is a subtly tasting super-cleansing juice bursting with fresh goodness.

ORANGE BLAST

210 calories per serving

Ingredients

- 1 orange
- 1 apple
- 1 carrot
- 1 tbsp fresh chopped basil
- Water

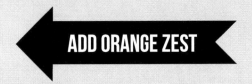

ADD ORANGE ZEST

Method

1 Rinse all the ingredients well.

2 Peel the orange and chop, discard the seeds.

3 Peel, core and chop the apple.

4 Top, tail, peel & chop the carrot.

5 Add the vegetables, fruit & basil to the bottle, making sure the ingredients do not go past the 600ml/20oz line on your bottle.

6 Top up with water, again being careful not to exceed the MAX line.

7 Twist on the blade and blend until smooth.

CHEFS NOTE
Adjust the quantity of fresh basil to suit your own taste.

REFRESHING LIME & CRANBERRY JUICE

295
calories per serving

···· *Ingredients* ····

- 2 apples
- 2 tbsp lime juice
- 200g/7oz fresh cranberries
- Water

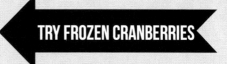
TRY FROZEN CRANBERRIES

···· *Method* ····

1 Rinse all the ingredients well.

2 Peel, core and chop the apples.

3 Add the fruit & lime juice to the bottle, making sure the ingredients do not go past the 600ml/20oz line on your bottle.

4 Top up with water, again being careful not to exceed the MAX line.

5 Twist on the blade and blend until smooth.

CHEFS NOTE
Adjust the quantity of lime juice to suit your own taste.

GOOD GRAPEFRUIT JUICE

220 calories per serving

Ingredients

- 1 pink grapefruit
- 200g/7oz pineapple chunks
- 2 tsp honey
- Water

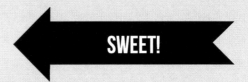
SWEET!

Method

1 Rinse all the ingredients well.

2 Peel and chop the grapefruit, discarding any seeds.

3 Add the fruit & honey to the bottle, making sure the ingredients do not go past the 600ml/20oz line on your bottle.

4 Top up with water, again being careful not to exceed the MAX line.

5 Twist on the blade and blend until smooth.

CHEFS NOTE
Good & Green: this is a simple and tasty morning juice.

FRUITY GRAPE JUICE

220
calories per
serving

Ingredients

- 1 handful of spinach
- 1 pear
- 200g/7oz green seedless grapes
- Water

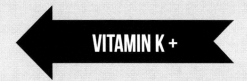

VITAMIN K +

Method

1 Rinse all the ingredients well.

2 Remove any thick, hard stems from the spinach and roughly chop.

3 Peel, core and chop the pear.

4 Remove the stalks from the grapes.

5 Add the vegetables & fruit to the bottle, making sure the ingredients do not go past the 600ml/20oz line on your bottle.

6 Top up with water, again being careful not to exceed the MAX line.

7 Twist on the blade and blend until smooth.

CHEFS NOTE
Red grapes are just as good in this juice.

FAST FRUIT SALAD

230 calories per serving

Ingredients

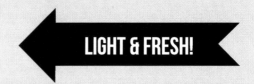

LIGHT & FRESH!

- **1** handful of spinach or spring greens
- **1** baby gem lettuce
- **1** banana
- **1** apple
- Water

Method

1 Rinse all the ingredients well.

2 Remove any thick, hard stems from the spinach and roughly chop.

3 Chop the lettuce, discard the heart.

4 Peel the banana and break into small pieces.

5 Peel, core and chop the apple.

6 Add the vegetables & fruit to the bottle, making sure the ingredients do not go past the 600ml/20oz line on your bottle.

7 Top up with water, again being careful not to exceed the MAX line.

8 Twist on the blade and blend until smooth.

CHEFS NOTE
Fast and fresh this is a lovely light juice.

SIMPLE STRAWBERRY SMOOTHIE

299 calories per serving

Ingredients

- 1 banana
- 200g/7oz strawberries
- 250ml/1 cup semi skimmed milk
- Water

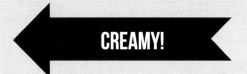

CREAMY!

Method

1 Rinse all the ingredients well.

2 Peel the banana and break into small pieces.

3 Cut the green tops of the strawberries and chop.

4 Add the fruit & milk to the bottle, making sure the ingredients do not go past the 600ml/20oz line on your bottle.

5 Top up with water if needed, again being careful not to exceed the MAX line.

6 Twist on the blade and blend until smooth.

CHEFS NOTE
Add more banana for extra creaminess.

MANGO BOOST JUICE

280 calories per serving

Ingredients

- 1 apple
- 200g/7oz mango
- 1 kiwi
- Water

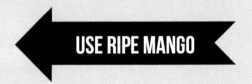

USE RIPE MANGO

Method

1 Rinse all the ingredients well.

2 Peel, core and chop the apple.

3 De-stone the mango and chop the flesh, discarding the rind.

4 Peel & chop the kiwi.

5 Add the fruit to the bottle, making sure the ingredients do not go past the 600ml/20oz line on your bottle.

6 Top up with water, again being careful not to exceed the MAX line.

7 Twist on the blade and blend until smooth.

CHEFS NOTE
Kiwi is an excellent source of vitamin 'C'.

HONEY & SWEET POTATO SMOOTHIE

285 calories per serving

Ingredients

- 1 apple
- 200g/7oz sweet potato
- 250ml/1 cup almond milk
- 2 tsp runny honey
- Water

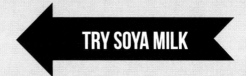

TRY SOYA MILK

Method

1 Rinse all the ingredients well.

2 Peel, core and chop the apple.

3 Peel and chop the sweet potato.

4 Add the vegetables, fruit & milk to the bottle, making sure the ingredients do not go past the 600ml/20oz line on your bottle.

5 Top up with water if it needs it, again being careful not to exceed the MAX line.

6 Twist on the blade and blend until smooth.

CHEFS NOTE
Adjust the honey and almond milk to suit your own taste.

PINEAPPLE & GINGER JUICE

210 calories per serving

Ingredients

- 1 tbsp lemon juice
- 1 banana
- 200g/7oz pineapple chunks
- 1 tsp grated fresh ginger root
- Water

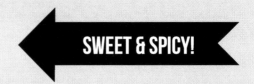

SWEET & SPICY!

Method

1 Rinse all the ingredients well.

2 Peel the banana and break into small pieces.

3 Add the fruit and lemon juice to the bottle, making sure the ingredients do not go past the 600ml/20oz line on your bottle.

4 Top up with water, again being careful not to exceed the MAX line.

5 Twist on the blade and blend until smooth.

CHEFS NOTE
Ginger has been used for centuries as a natural treatment for coughs and colds.

ICY FRUIT CHARD

240 calories per serving

Ingredients

- 1 small handful Swiss chard leaves
- 1 banana
- 200g/7oz fresh pineapple chunks
- Water
- Handful of ice

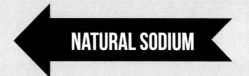

NATURAL SODIUM

Method

1 Rinse all the ingredients well.

2 Roughly chop the chard leaves..

3 Peel the banana and break into small pieces.

4 Chop the pineapple and add all the fruit & salad to the bottle, making sure the ingredients do not go past the 600ml/20oz line on your bottle.

5 Top up with water & ice, again being careful not to exceed the MAX line.

6 Twist on the blade and blend until smooth.

CHEFS NOTE
Try using spinach if you find chard a little bitter.

CITRUS ALMOND MILK

250 calories per serving

Ingredients

- 1 orange
- 200g/7oz mixed berries
- 250ml/1 cup almond milk
- 2 tsp honey
- 25g/1oz fresh walnuts
- Water

Method

1 Rinse all the ingredients well.

2 Peel the orange and roughly chop (discard any seeds).

3 Add the fruit, milk, honey & walnuts to the bottle, making sure the ingredients do not go past the 600ml/20oz line on your bottle.

4 Top up with water if needed, again being careful not to exceed the MAX line.

5 Twist on the blade and blend until smooth.

CHEFS NOTE

Chop the walnuts before blending for a smooth finish.

CREAMY COCONUT JUICE

275 calories per serving

Ingredients

- 1 apple
- 1 banana
- 250ml/1 cup coconut water
- ½ tsp ground cinnamon
- Water

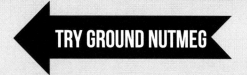

TRY GROUND NUTMEG

Method

1 Rinse all the ingredients well.

2 Peel, core and dice the apple.

3 Peel the banana and break into small pieces.

4 Add the fruit & coconut water to the bottle, making sure the ingredients do not go past the 600ml/20oz line on your bottle.

5 Top up with water if needed, again being careful not to exceed the MAX line.

6 Twist on the blade and blend until smooth.

CHEFS NOTE
Try adding tablespoon of coconut cream if you want a richer blend.

PINEAPPLE & COCONUT WATER

255
calories per serving

Ingredients

- 1 banana
- 200g/7oz fresh pineapple
- 250ml/1 cup coconut water
- Water

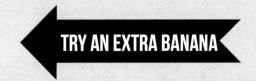

TRY AN EXTRA BANANA

Method

1 Rinse all the ingredients well.

2 Peel the banana and break into small pieces.

3 Add the fruit & coconut water to the bottle, making sure the ingredients do not go past the 600ml/20oz line on your bottle.

4 Top up with water if needed, again being careful not to exceed the MAX line.

5 Twist on the blade and blend until smooth.

CHEFS NOTE
Try adding two tablespoons of acai berries to this blend for extra goodness.

BANANA OATS

235
calories per
serving

Ingredients

- 1 banana
- 1 apple
- 2 tbsp rolled oats
- Water

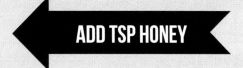
ADD TSP HONEY

Method

1 Rinse all the ingredients well.

2 Peel the banana and break into small pieces.

3 Peel, core and cube the apple.

4 Add the fruit, & oats to the bottle, making sure the ingredients do not go past the 600ml/20oz line on your bottle.

5 Top up with water, again being careful not to exceed the MAX line.

6 Twist on the blade and blend until smooth.

CHEFS NOTE
This is a lovely cleansing blend, great at breakfast time.

MANGO & KIWI JUICE

255
calories per
serving

Ingredients

- 1 kiwi fruit
- 150g/5oz fresh mango
- 1 banana
- Water

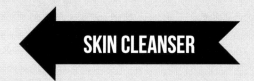

SKIN CLEANSER

Method

1 Rinse all the ingredients well.

2 Peel & dice the kiwi.

3 De-stone, peel and chop the mango.

4 Peel the banana and break into small pieces.

5 Add the fruit to the bottle, making sure the ingredients do not go past the 600ml/20oz line on your bottle.

6 Top up with water, again being careful not to exceed the MAX line.

7 Twist on the blade and blend until smooth.

CHEFS NOTE

Try making this blend using soya milk instead of water as the base.

THE *Skinny*

BLEND ›*ACTIVE*

LEAN BODY
YOGA WORKOUT PLAN

SMOOTHIES & JUICES UNDER 400 CALORIES

SUPER SMOOTH STRAWBERRIES

SERVES 1

375 calories per serving

Ingredients

- 200g/7oz strawberries
- ½ ripe avocado
- 250ml/1 cup almond milk
- Water

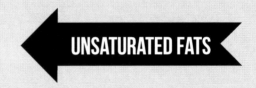

UNSATURATED FATS

Method

1 Rinse all the ingredients well.

2 Remove the stalks and chop the strawberries.

3 De-stone the avocado and scoop out the flesh, remove the rind.

4 Add the fruit, avocado & almond milk to the bottle, making sure the ingredients do not go past the 600ml/20oz line on your bottle.

5 Top up with water if needed, again being careful not to exceed the MAX line.

6 Twist on the blade and blend until smooth.

CHEFS NOTE
Raspberries are also good in this smoothie.

NUTTY BLUEBERRY SMOOTHIE

310 calories per serving

Ingredients

- 200g/7oz blueberries
- 1 banana
- 1 tbsp ground almonds
- 250ml/1 cup almond milk
- Water

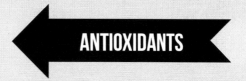

ANTIOXIDANTS

Method

1 Rinse all the ingredients well.

2 Peel the banana and break into small pieces.

3 Add the fruit, milk & ground almonds to the bottle, making sure the ingredients do not go past the 600ml/20oz line on your bottle.

4 Top up with water if it needs it, again being careful not to exceed the MAX line.

5 Twist on the blade and blend until smooth.

CHEFS NOTE
In place of ground almonds try freshly chopped walnuts.

PROTEIN POWER SMOOTHIE

SERVES 1

360 calories per serving

Ingredients

- 1 banana
- 1 scoop protein powder
- 1 tbsp low fat peanut butter
- 250ml/1 cup almond milk
- Water

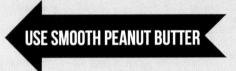

USE SMOOTH PEANUT BUTTER

Method

1 Peel the banana and break into small pieces.

2 Add all the ingredients to the bottle, making sure the contents do not go past the 600ml/20oz line on your bottle.

3 Twist on the blade and blend until smooth.

CHEFS NOTE

Most protein powder comes with a measuring scoop. If not just use one level tablespoon of powder.

NUTTY CHOCOLATE PROTEIN SMOOTHIE

375 calories per serving

Ingredients

- 1 banana
- 1 scoop protein powder
- 1 tbsp hazelnut chocolate spread
- 250ml/1 cup semi-skimmed milk

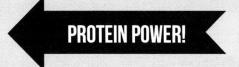

PROTEIN POWER!

Method

1 Peel the banana and break into small pieces.

2 Add all the ingredients to the bottle, making sure the contents do not go past the 600ml/20oz line on your bottle.

3 Twist on the blade and blend until smooth.

CHEFS NOTE

Nutella is a great hazelnut chocolate spread but any variety will work fine.

CINNAMON PEACH SMOOTHIE

390
calories per serving

Ingredients

- 1 peach
- 1 apple
- 1 banana

- 250ml/1 cup semi skimmed milk
- Pinch of ground cinnamon
- Water

Method

1 Rinse all the ingredients well.

2 Peel, de-stone and chop the peach

3 Peel, core & chop the apple.

4 Peel the banana and break into small pieces.

5 Add the fruit, milk & cinnamon to the bottle, making sure the ingredients do not go past the 600ml/20oz line on your bottle.

6 Top up with water if it needs it, again being careful not to exceed the MAX line.

7 Twist on the blade and blend until smooth.

CHEFS NOTE
Unsweetened tinned peaches will work just fine in place of fresh peaches.

DOUBLE ALMOND & MANGO SMOOTHIE

355 calories per serving

Ingredients

- 1 mango
- 1 banana
- 250ml/1 cup almond milk
- 1 tbsp ground almonds
- Water

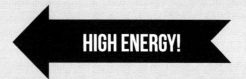

HIGH ENERGY!

Method

1 Peel, de-stone and chop the mango.

2 Peel the banana and break into small pieces.

3 Add the fruit, milk & ground almonds to the bottle, making sure the ingredients do not go past the 600ml/20oz line on your bottle.

4 Top up with water if it needs it, again being careful not to exceed the MAX line.

5 Twist on the blade and blend until smooth.

CHEFS NOTE
You could easily use fresh chopped almonds in place of ground almonds.

BANANA NUT SMOOTHIE

330
calories per serving

Ingredients

- 2 bananas
- 1 tbsp low fat smooth peanut butter
- 1 cup/250ml almond milk

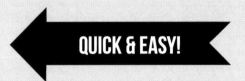

QUICK & EASY!

Method

1 Peel the banana and break into small pieces.

2 Add the bananas, peanut butter & almond milk to the bottle, making sure the ingredients do not go past the 600ml/20oz line on your bottle.

3 Twist on the blade and blend until smooth.

CHEFS NOTE
Use smooth peanut butter rather than the crunchy variety.

STRAWBERRY & PEANUT SMOOTHIE

385 calories per serving

Ingredients

- 200g/7oz strawberries
- 1 banana
- 1 tbsp smooth peanut butter
- 1 cup/250ml semi skimmed milk

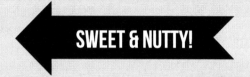

SWEET & NUTTY!

Method

1 Remove the green tops and chop the strawberries.

2 Peel the banana and break into small pieces

3 Add the strawberries, banana, peanut butter & milk to the bottle, making sure the ingredients do not go past the 600ml/20oz line on your bottle.

4 Twist on the blade and blend until smooth.

CHEFS NOTE
Soya milk or almond milk will also work well in this smoothie.

AVOCADO & APPLE BLEND

280 calories per serving

---- Ingredients ----

- ½ ripe avocado
- 1 apple
- 2 mint leaves
- 1 tsp lime juice
- Water

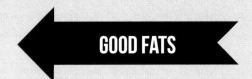

GOOD FATS

---- Method ----

1 Rinse all the ingredients well.

2 De-stone the avocado and scoop out the flesh, discard the rind.

3 Peel, core and chop the apple.

4 Add the fruit, mint & lime jiuce to the bottle, making sure the ingredients do not go past the 600ml/20oz line on your bottle.

5 Top up with water, again being careful not to exceed the MAX line.

6 Twist on the blade and blend until smooth.

CHEFS NOTE
Creamy and light this blend is also good with a touch of spice. Try adding some freshly ground black pepper.

CREAMY GREEN SMOOTHIE

370 calories per serving

Ingredients

- 1 handful of spinach
- ½ ripe avocado
- 1 apple
- 250ml/1 cup soya milk
- Water

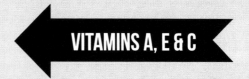

VITAMINS A, E & C

Method

1 Rinse all the ingredients well.

2 Remove any thick, hard stems from the spinach and roughly chop.

3 De-stone the avocado and scoop out the flesh, discard the rind.

4 Peel, core and chop the apple.

5 Add the fruit, vegetables & soya milk to the bottle, making sure the ingredients do not go past the 600ml/20oz line on your bottle.

6 Top up with water if needed, again being careful not to exceed the MAX line.

7 Twist on the blade and blend until smooth.

CHEFS NOTE

Try substituting the spinach for kale if you want some 'hardcore' greens.

BANANA & CHIA SEED SMOOTHIE

315 calories per serving

Ingredients

- 2 bananas
- 1 tsp chia seeds
- 250ml/1 cup almond milk
- Water

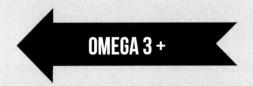

OMEGA 3 +

Method

1 Rinse all the ingredients well.

2 Peel the bananas and break into small pieces.

3 Add the bananas, chia seeds & almond milk to the bottle, making sure the ingredients do not go past the 600ml/20oz line on your bottle.

4 Top up with water if it needs it, again being careful not to exceed the MAX line.

5 Twist on the blade and blend until smooth.

CHEFS NOTE

Chia seeds are now widely available, they are packed with nutrients.

BREAKFAST OAT SMOOTHIE

395 calories per serving

Ingredients

- 2 bananas
- 1 tbsp rolled oats
- 1 tbsp honey
- 250ml/1 cup soya milk
- Water

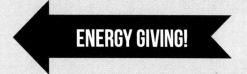

ENERGY GIVING!

Method

1 Rinse all the ingredients well.

2 Peel the bananas and break into small pieces.

3 Add the bananas, oats, honey & soya milk to the bottle, making sure the ingredients do not go past the 600ml/20oz line on your bottle.

4 Top up with water if it needs it, again being careful not to exceed the MAX line.

5 Twist on the blade and blend until smooth.

CHEFS NOTE
You can add some chopped apple or pear to this smoothie too if you like.

CASHEW PEACH SMOOTHIE

SERVES 1

370 calories per serving

Ingredients

- 1 banana
- 2 peaches
- 50g/2oz cashew nuts
- 250ml/1 cup almond milk
- Water

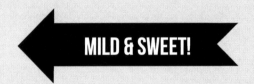
MILD & SWEET!

Method

1 Rinse all the ingredients well.

2 Peel the banana and break into small pieces.

3 Peel, de-stone and chop the peaches.

4 Chop the cashew nuts.

5 Add the fruit, nuts & almond milk to the bottle, making sure the ingredients do not go past the 600ml/20oz line on your bottle.

6 Top up with water if it needs it, again being careful not to exceed the MAX line.

7 Twist on the blade and blend until smooth.

CHEFS NOTE
Tinned peaches will work just as well if you don't have time to peel fresh peaches.

GOJI BERRY SMOOTHIE

340 calories per serving

Ingredients

- 1 banana
- 200g/7oz strawberries
- 1 tbsp goji berries
- 250ml/1 cup almond milk
- Water

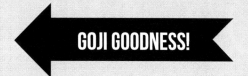
GOJI GOODNESS!

Method

1 Rinse all the ingredients well.

2 Peel the banana and break into small pieces.

3 Remove the green tops from the strawberries and chop.

4 Add the fruit & almond milk to the bottle, making sure the ingredients do not go past the 600ml/20oz line on your bottle.

5 Top up with water if needed, again being careful not to exceed the MAX line.

6 Twist on the blade and blend until smooth.

CHEFS NOTE

Recent studies have indicated that goji berries may help protect against the influenza virus.

BLUEBERRY & AVOCADO JUICE

375 calories per serving

Ingredients

- ½ ripe avocado
- 1 banana
- 200g/7oz blueberries
- 2 tsp honey
- Water

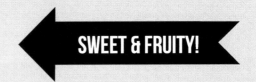

SWEET & FRUITY!

Method

1 Rinse all the ingredients well.

2 De-stone the avocado and scoop out the flesh, discard the rind.

3 Peel the banana and break into small pieces.

4 Add the fruit, avocado & honey to the bottle, making sure the ingredients do not go past the 600ml/20oz line on your bottle.

5 Top up with water, again being careful not to exceed the MAX line.

6 Twist on the blade and blend until smooth.

CHEFS NOTE
You can use any type of sweet berry you prefer.

YOGA *Workouts*

We recommend trying to find the time to practice yoga every day. A daily session will boost physical & mental wellbeing. The three workouts which have been developed in this book can be undertaken any time of the day depending on your schedule - although you will find the Morning & Tummy Toning Yoga most suited to the day time (or when you need to be refreshed) whilst the restful sleep yoga is best suited for the very the end of the day.

The first two workouts will take around 15 minutes to complete. The third is a 30 minute relaxation session. All you need to get started is a mat, a block and pillows for support. That said there is no need to run out and buy any equipment at all. You can do any of these routines comfortably on a rug or carpet and the yoga block can be substituted for a small strong shoe sized box.

Yoga should never be approached as a competitive sport. It is a personal journey. Always listen to your body and never push yourself too hard. Concentrating on breathing is an extremely important part of yoga practice and you will learnt to use the rhythm of your breathing to help you move through the poses. Always move into poses on a breath exhalation and make sure you move slowly and methodically. Try to relax your facial muscles and jaw whilst tensing the muscles you should be concentrating on.

Restful Sleep Workout Tips:

When you are undertaking this workout try to concentrate on nothing other than your own breathing. Try not to alter it but instead just feel it's natural rhythm and depth. Inevitably your mind will jump around from thought to thought - seemingly uncontrollably. Try not to become frustrated by this. Instead notice where your mind is and each time gently bring your thoughts back to your breathing. This is a skill in itself and it won't come right away. Emptying your mind is not as easy as it sounds, but have patience with yourself. If you try to anchor your thoughts around your breathing and repeat this routine regularly you will learn to calm your mind and move towards a stillness which will benefit your long term well-being.

Morning YOGA

- Pose 1: **COW**
- Pose 2: **CAT**
- Pose 3: **COBRA**
- Pose 4: **EXTENSION**
- Pose 5: **ELBOW TO KNEE**
- Pose 6: **BIND**
- Pose 7: **LOW LUNGE**

- Pose 8: **LOW LUNGE STRETCH**
- Pose 9: **LIZARD POSE**
- Pose 10: **HALF SPLITS**
- Pose 11: **TWISTED MONKEY**
- Pose 12: **SIDE PLANK**
- Pose 13: **MOUNTAIN POSE**

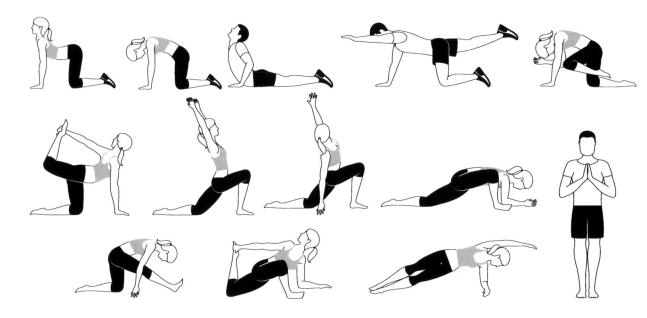

We have called this workout Morning Yoga as it is a wonderful routine to wake up with, but it can be used at any time throughout the day to refresh your mood and perk you up. It will take no more than 15 minutes and will prepare you for whatever lies ahead.

Cow

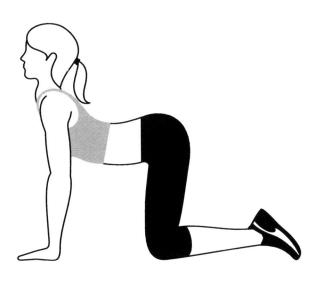

Come onto your hands and knees with hips placed over the knees. Shoulders positioned over the wrists. Your knees and hands should be shoulder distance apart, and the spine neutral. On exhalation gently lift your tail bone up to the sky, let your belly drop toward the mat and look up. Hold for a few moments before going into the next pose.

Cat

On a breath exhalation, lengthen your tail bone to the ground, draw the belly up to the spine and round the upper back like a cat. Concentrate on pressing your hands into the mat to open the shoulder blades. Let the head drop. Gently and slowly move through ten rounds of Cat/Cow, then return to a neutral spine.

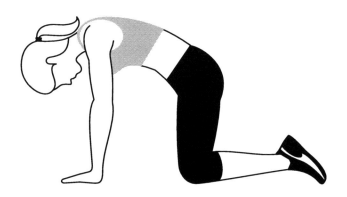

Cobra

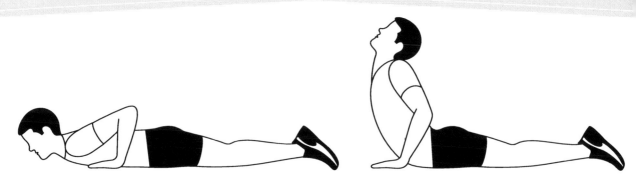

Lie face-down on mat. With elbows bent place the palms on each side of your body in line with the breastbone. Come onto fingertips and point elbows toward sky and out to sides. Press your pelvis, toes, and fingertips into the mat. On exhalation straighten the arms enough to fully lift the chest off the mat. Keep the spine long and tip the head back. Hold for 8 full deep breaths, engaging the thighs, before relaxing back onto the mat.

Extension

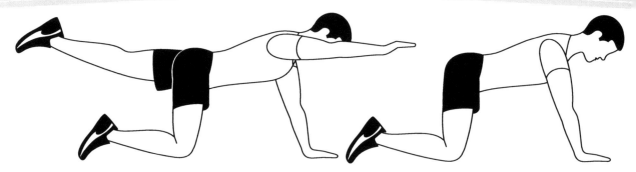

Move onto all fours. Lift your left leg and extend behind you whilst reaching your right arm forward. Lengthen your spine as you extend the arm and leg in opposite directions. Engage the core and maintain length in the back of the neck as you gaze down just in front of your hand on the mat. Hold for 5 long deep breaths. Reverse position and repeat.

Elbow To KNEE

From the extension pose move into the next pose by bringing your left elbow and your right knee in together to touch under the body. Do this on an exhalation and engage the core as you do so. Inhale to fully extend arm and leg into the extension pose and exhale to bring elbow and knee to touch. Repeat this in a careful measured way 5 times. Return to all fours ready for the next pose. Reverse position and repeat.

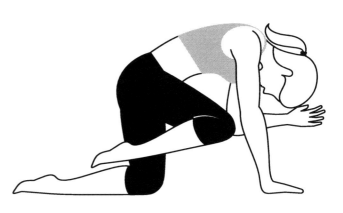

Bind

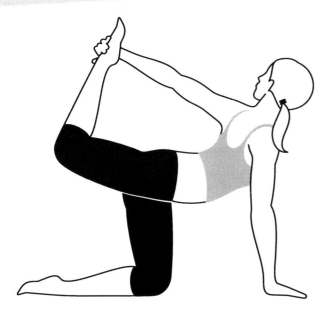

Reach left arm behind you and take hold of the right foot. Point the toes of this foot to the sky. Rolling the left shoulder toward the sky and draw the right shoulder back and down away from the right ear. Extend straight back from the hip. Hold for 5 slow deep breaths. Release from the pose. Lie on your back, hug knees to chest and gently rock side to side a few times to release the back. Reverse position and repeat.

Low LUNGE

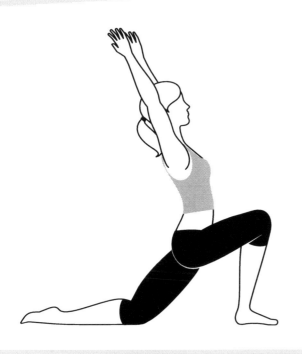

Stand straight on the mat with arms by sides. Step your right foot forward in between your hands, and on exhalation reach your arms up to the sky, keeping shoulders away from the ears. Push your right foot down and lower your hips towards the mat. Engage the core whilst avoiding puffing out the chest. Look forwards to the sky and hold the pose for 5 slow deep breaths. Reverse position and repeat.

Low Lunge STRETCH

From low lunge, reach your right fingertips down to the ground (you may wish to use a block). Exhale and reach up with the left fingertips for a full stretch. Concentrate on balance by pressing the right foot down into the mat. Look skywards but do not force your neck if this is uncomfortable. Keep the core engaged and the chest open. Feel the length of the stretch through your body and hold for 5 slow deep breaths. Reverse position and repeat.

Lizard POSE

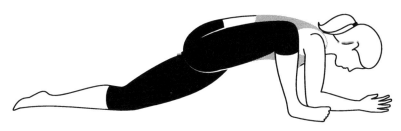

Move onto all fours on the mat. Bend the right knee and place the sole of the right foot into to the mat. On exhalation lower your body weight down to your forearms with palms facing each other. Move shoulders down away from the ears. Relax the right knee and allow it to rotate in the hip joint so that the knee falls to the right and the right foot is on its outer right edge. Do not force your knee down. Hold for 5 slow deep breaths before releasing from the pose. Reverse position and repeat.

Half SPLITS

Return to all fours. On exhalation slowly pull your hips back so that they are positioned over your left knee whilst straightening the right leg, Press your right heel into the mat, lengthen the right leg and flex the toes of the right foot back towards you. Keep the neck straight and look to the floor. Engage the core and hold for 5 slow deep breaths. Reverse position and repeat.

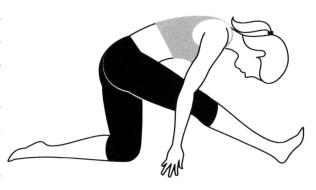

Twisted MONKEY

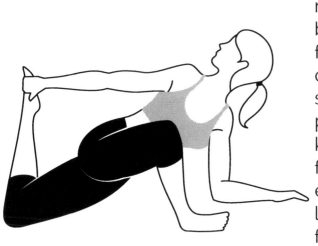

Return to all fours. On exhalation reach the right arm up and then back to take hold of your left foot. Roll the right shoulder back opening the chest. The left forearm should be flat on the mat with the palm extended. Allow the right knee to gently drop towards the floor as you come onto the outer edge of your right foot. Carefully lean the upper body back and hold for 5 slow deep breaths. Reverse position and repeat.

Side PLANK

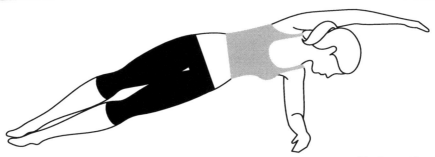

From Twisted Monkey moving your left forearm parallel to the top of the mat. Straighten the legs so that they rest on top of each other. Engage the core, extend the left arm over your head and lift the weight of your body to move into the side plank position. Feel the stretch through the side body and hold for 5 slow deep breaths. If you need stability split your legs so that both feet touch the floor. Reverse position and repeat.

Mountain POSE

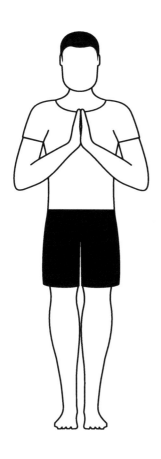

Finish the session with Mountain Pose by standing straight with legs and feet together, heels slightly apart, and arms at sides with palms facing forward. Keep your spine long, shoulders rolled back and away from the ears, spread the toes and press soles of the feet into mat. Engage thighs and lower belly, bring the gaze of the eyes towards the floor some distance ahead of you and lightly close the eyes. Slowly bring hands together at the centre of the chest and hold for 10 long deep breaths.

Tummy Toning YOGA

- Pose 1: **MOUNTAIN POSE**
- Pose 2: **STANDING LEAN**
- Pose 3: **COBRA**
- Pose 4: **MOUNTAIN CHAIR**
- Pose 5: **WARRIOR POSE**

- Pose 6: **CHEST OPENER**
- Pose 7: **DOWNWARD DOG**
- Pose 8: **PARTIAL PLANK**
- Pose 9: **PARTIAL SIDE PLANK**

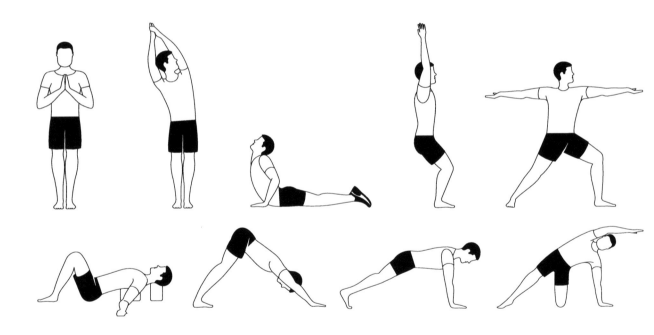

This routine is ideal for helping to tighten your core and it's also good for the thighs. Each of the poses will encourage you to use many of the core muscles we often forget about and should take no more than 15 minutes.

Mountain POSE

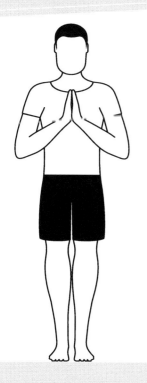

Begin the session with this iconic yoga pose by standing straight with legs and feet together, heels slightly apart, and arms at sides with palms facing forward. Keep your spine long, shoulders rolled back and away from the ears, spread the toes and press soles of the feet into mat. Engage thighs and core, bring the gaze of the eyes towards the floor some distance ahead of you and lightly close the eyes. Slowly bring hands together at the centre of the chest and hold for 10 long deep breaths.

Standing LEAN

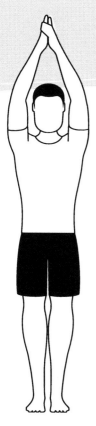

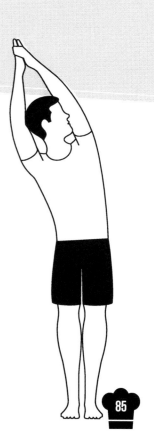

Begin by gently joining the palms above the head with the arms straight. Squeeze the inner arms in toward the ears but keep the shoulders down away from the ears. On your breath exhalation, press feet down, engage thighs and core, and stretch up and evenly over to right. Repeat the pose this time on the left side. Remember to engage the core and thighs each time and move on exhalation. Do this slowly on each side 4 times.

Cobra

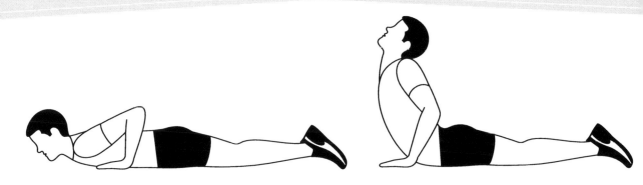

Lie face-down on mat. With elbows bent place the palms on each side of your body in line with the breastbone. Come onto fingertips and point elbows toward sky and out to sides. Press your pelvis, toes, and fingertips into the mat. On exhalation straighten the arms enough to fully lift the chest off the mat. Keep the spine long and tip the head back. Hold for 8 full deep breaths, engaging the core & thighs, before relaxing back onto the mat.

Mountain CHAIR

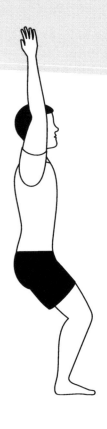

Stand straight with arms above the head and palms facing each other. On exhalation, sweep arms down and behind your body, bending knees and lowering hips. Inhale and reach arms overhead, biceps by ears with palms turned in toward each other, and sit into chair pose strongly engaging the core. On your next exhalation return to start. Repeat 10 times in a slow measured way.

Warrior POSE

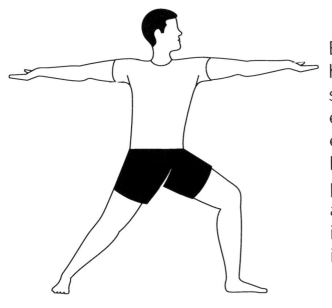

Extend the arms out at shoulder height and step your feet apart so they are positioned below the extended wrists. Have the outer edge of back foot parallel to back of mat and toes of front foot pointing forward. Engage the core and slowly bend front knee, lining it up over front ankle, and come into warrior pose with palms up.

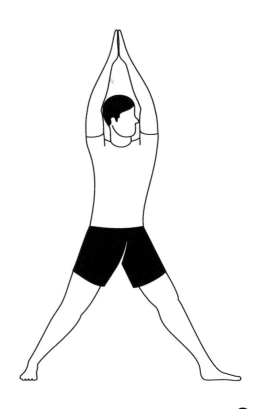

On exhalation, straighten your front leg and sweep the arms overhead, bringing palms together . On inhalation, return to warrior pose. Repeat 8 times. Switch legs and repeat.

Chest OPENER

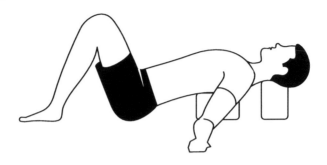

Lie face-up on mat with knees bent and feet positioned hip-width apart. Place a yoga block beneath your head and another lengthwise between shoulder blades. Bring arms out to sides and allow your chest to open. Engage your core strongly. Breathe through your stretch and stay in this pose for 2 minutes.

Downward DOG

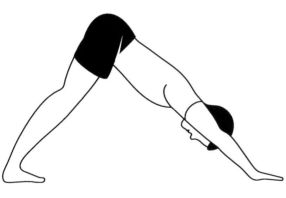

Start on all fours with knees and hands hip-width apart . Curl the feet to push toes into mat. On exhalation push down into hands and feet. Engage the core strongly and lift hips to sky keeping the back straight as if you are trying to push the mat away from yourself with your hands. Press down strongly through arms and balls of feet and lower heels onto the mat (don't worry if you have to bend your knees a little). Hold for 5 deep breaths keeping the core and thighs engaged throughout.

Partial PLANK

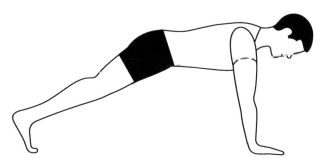

From Downward Dog, exhale and bring your body forward to come into the pose. Lengthen your spine and press heels towards the back of the room, engaging your core and thighs. Hold this position for a few moments then on exhalation, push down back into the downward dog pose. Keep the core and thighs engaged as you repeat this slowly 7 times.

Partial Side PLANK

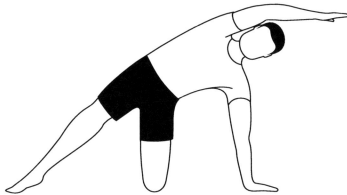

Move onto your knees. Extend the right leg whilst the left stays rooted to the floor. On exhalation turn your body to the right, shifting your weight onto left palm and right foot. Keep your spine and neck in line as you extend the right arm overhead, with palm facing down. Hold for 8 full deep breaths. Repeat on opposite side.

Restful Sleep YOGA

- Pose 1: **COW**
- Pose 2: **CAT**
- Pose 3: **BRIDGE POSE**
- Pose 4: **LEGS UP THE WALL**
- Pose 5: **SEATED FORWARD BEND**
- Pose 6: **WIDE LEG FORWARD BEND**
- Pose 7: **COBRA**
- Pose 8: **LEFT NOSTRIL BREATHING**

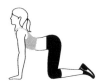 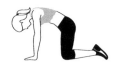 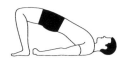

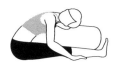 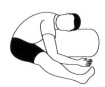 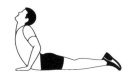

This gentle routine is ideal for preparing for bed, winding down in the evening or if you wish to meditate/rest throughout the day. You will need to have a mat and some pillows to hand and it should take no more than 30 minutes. Feel free to lengthen or shorten each of the poses to suit your own schedule.

Cow

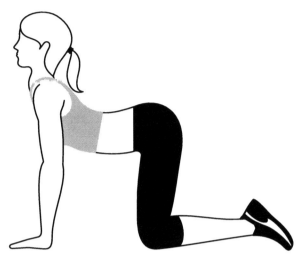

Come onto your hands and knees with hips placed over the knees. Shoulders positioned over the wrists. Your knees and hands should be shoulder distance apart, and the spine neutral. On exhalation gently lift your tail bone up to the sky, let your belly drop toward the mat and look up. Hold for a few moments before going into the next pose.

Cat

On a breath exhalation, lengthen your tail bone to the ground, draw the belly up to the spine and round the upper back like a cat. Concentrate on pressing your hands into the mat to open the shoulder blades. Let the head drop. Gently and slowly move through ten rounds of Cat/Cow, then return to a neutral spine.

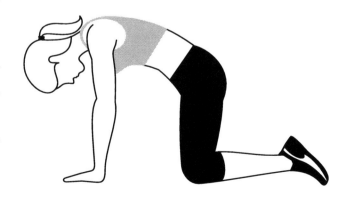

Bridge POSE

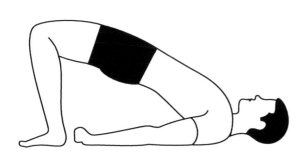

On your mat lie down with feet flat on the floor hip-width apart. Place your hands beside you with palms facing down. Engage your thighs and core and on exhalation lift your body up so that your back is flat and your knees are at a 45 degree angle whilst your arms remain flat on the floor. Settle into the pose and hold it for 2-3 minutes if you can.

Legs Up THE WALL

Position yourself on your mat side-on close up to wall. Roll onto your back with your legs up in the air. Twist yourself around 90 degrees so that your legs rest straight up against the wall. Shuffle your bottom up tight against the wall if you need to. Keep your arms straight by your side with the palms flat down. Remain in this pose for 5 minutes breathing deeply and slowly, concentrating on nothing other than movement and feeling of your breath.

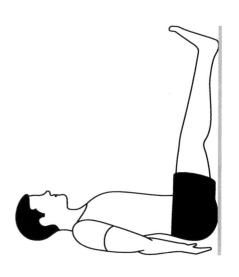

Seated Forward BEND

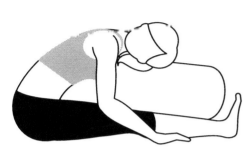

Sit on the mat with your legs straight out in front of you. Place pillow(s) on your thighs against your stomach (you may need to experiment with the height of the support). Put your arms above your head then reach forward as you bend your body onto the pillow and rest the side of your head onto the pillow support. Allow your arms to rest by your side and remain in this position for 5 minutes.

Wide Leg Forward BEND

This is a variation on the last pose. This time move your legs apart whilst you are in an upright sitting position. Place your cushion(s) onto the floor between your legs. Put your arms above your head then reach forward as you bend your body onto the pillow and rest the side of your head onto the pillow support – use the opposite side of your head from the last pose. Allow your arms to rest by your side and remain in this position for 5 minutes. If this feels uncomfortable it can be helpful to sit on a block or cushion to lift your pelvis or/and you may wish to bend your knees a little.

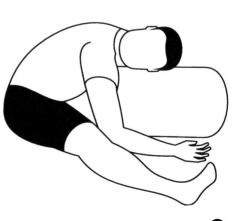

Cobra

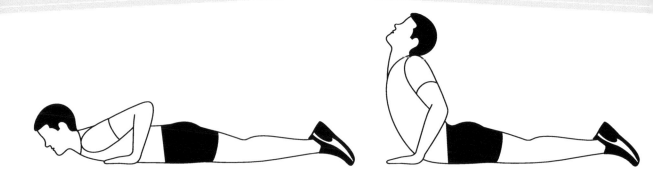

Lie face-down on mat. With elbows bent place palms a little away from each side of your body in line with the breastbone. Come onto fingertips and point elbows toward sky and out to sides Press pelvis, toes, and fingertips into floor. On exhalation straighten the arms enough to lift the chest off the mat. Keep the spine long and tip the head back. Hold for 8 full deep breaths before relaxing back onto the mat.

Left Nostril BREATHING

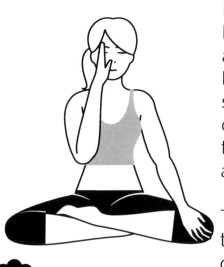

Sit in a comfortable cross- legged position. Keep your back straight with your shoulders low down away from your ears. Try to imagine a piece of string being pulled from above lifting the crown of your head up towards the sky. Cover your right nostril with your thumb or finger and begin breathing in and out through your left nostril. Breathe like this for at least 2 minutes.

This may seem strange but breathing through the left nostril has a calming effect on the nervous system and aids mediation and restful sleep.

Other
COOKNATION
TITLES

If you enjoyed **The** *Skinny* **Blend Active Lean Body Yoga Workout Plan** you may also be interested in other *Skinny* titles in the CookNation series.

Visit **www.bellmackenzie.com** to browse the full catalogue.

18442266R00055

Printed in Great Britain
by Amazon